# The Baby Puree Cookbook

Puree Recipes for Grown-ups and Weaning

BY

MOLLY MILLS

Copyright © 2019 by Molly Mills

# License Notes

No part of this book may be copied, replicated, distributed, sold or shared without the express and written consent of the Author.

The ideas expressed in the book are for entertainment purposes. The Reader assumes all risk when following any guidelines and the Author accepts no responsibility if damages occur due to actions taken by the Reader.

# Table of Contents

Introduction .................................................................. 6

Swede Purée ................................................................. 8

Baked Pumpkin Puree .................................................... 10

Serrouda - Moroccan Chickpea Puree (Appetizer, Side, Dip) ................................................................................ 12

Pan-Fried Scallops with Parsnip Purée & Pancetta Crumbs ................................................................................ 15

Greek Fava Split Pea Puree ............................................ 19

Smoked Aubergine Purée ............................................... 21

Creamy Corn Soup ......................................................... 23

Strawberry Puree ............................................................ 26

Carrot & Star Anise Purée .............................................. 28

Bacon-Wrapped Scallops with Corn Puree ..................... 31

Herb-Crusted Rack of Lamb With The White Bean Purée' ................................................................... 35

Slow Cooker Creamy Corn Chowder ............................ 39

Cauliflower Puree ............................................................ 41

Pea Puree ........................................................................... 43

Potato Puree ...................................................................... 45

Puree Meals for Babies ....................................................... 47

Spinach, Sweet Potato & Yellow Split Pea Purée ......... 48

Cauliflower Cheese Purée ............................................... 50

Carrot, Celeriac & Apple Purée ..................................... 52

Haddock, Cauliflower & Potato Purée ......................... 54

Apple & Beetroot Purée .................................................. 56

Salmon, Pea & Potato Purée ........................................... 58

Carrot and Red Lentil Puree ........................................... 60

Roasted Butternut Squash and Garlic Purée ................ 62

Banana and Avocado Puree ............................................ 64

Spiced Pear Purée ............................................................... 66

Rice Puree and Spiced Carrot ............................................ 68

Mango Blueberry Puree with A Splash Of Milk ........... 70

Banana Puree & Roast Pear ............................................... 71

Apple Walnut Puree ............................................................ 73

Banana and Strawberry Puree .......................................... 75

Conclusion ................................................................................ 77

About the Author .................................................................... 78

Don't Miss Out! ....................................................................... 80

# Introduction

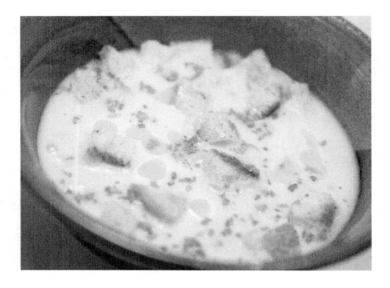

If for some reason you cannot eat solid food, then pureed food are your next best options. This fact is known for babies as they have not developed the facilities to chew food before they swallow. For adults, the need for puree food is usually caused by health concern or injury that inhibits their ability to chew, swallow, and digest properly. However, pureed food is not exclusive to babies and the category of adults highlighted above, some grownups just love the taste and texture of pureed food, and who can blame them?

Whatever your reasons for pureed food are, this book has you covered. A pureed diet gives you more variety and nutrients, anyway, and they are easier to swallow and digest. The primary objective of this book is to ensure that you have a collection of food to satisfy your nutritional needs and prevent any form of malnutrition.

This book is divided into two sections; one section for pureed food for adults, featuring appetizers, side dishes and mains, and the other section for babies. Shall we begin now?

Oh, wait, you need a food processor or blender to make most of these recipes. You have either of the two already? Great! Now, let us begin.

# Swede Purée

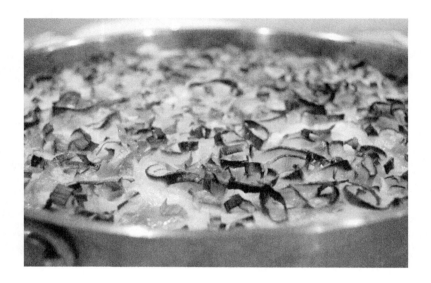

This puree is the ideal comfort food, especially on cold nights. It combines well with casseroles, stews, and ragus to give you something to smile about and look forward to making. Now, let's get to making it.

**Total Cooking Time:** 30 minutes

**Serving Size:** 4

**Ingredients:**

- 2 tbsp natural yogurt
- 1 swede (peeled and chopped)
- Parsley (chopped)
- 3 tbsp butter
- Salt

**Instructions:**

1. Dump the swede in a pan and top with boiling water. Put 1 tablespoon salt and bring to a boil. Let it cook for 20 minutes or until soft.

2. When the swede becomes soft, drain to remove the water. Put in a food processor and add butter and yogurt. Now, leave the processor to do its work.

3. Serve into plates and garnish with the parsley.

# Baked Pumpkin Puree

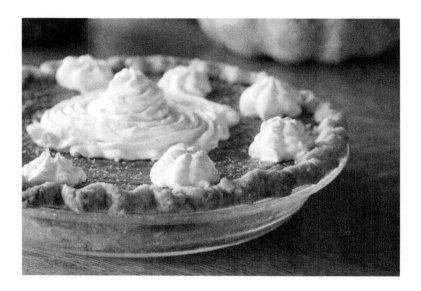

If you love pumpkin meals, you would know that a lot of them require the use of pumpkin puree. Now, here is the good news; you will easily find them in cans at the store or supermarket. But there is much better news; you can make them all by yourself at home; they are easy to make, anyway. So, when there is an abundance of pumpkin, why don't you make them into a puree and save yourself some money? By the way, they make for excellent side dishes and desserts too.

**Total Cooking Time:** 55 minutes

**Serving Size:** 8

**Ingredients:**

- 1 fresh pumpkin (Should be in the region of 3-5 lbs.)
- 1/2 cup water

**Instructions:**

1. Preheat oven to 350 F.

2. Cut out the top of the pumpkin with a knife. Remove the fibrous layer and the seeds. After this, slice the pumpkin into sizeable pieces.

3. Put the pumpkin in a pan and top with 1/2 cup water. Now, wrap the opening of the pan with a foil.

4. Put in the oven and bake from 50 minutes to 1 hour, or until pumpkin is tender (you can determine this by sticking a fork into a piece of pumpkin.)

5. Leave it to cool down to prevent burning yourself. Now, cut the soft pulp from the skin and put in a food processor. Pulse till you get your smooth puree.

N.B: Heat it if you are eating it immediately and put leftovers in the fridge. Ensure that you consume within 3 days.

# Serrouda - Moroccan Chickpea Puree (Appetizer, Side, Dip)

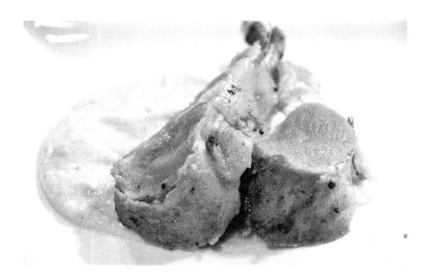

Chickpeas feature prominently in the Moroccan gastronomy. They also make a great puree, as you will find in this recipe. Here is how it happens; the dried chickpeas are first soaked, then they are peeled. Afterward, they are cooked to soften, then before they go through a food processor to transform into the puree.

It's a process you would enjoy, trust me.

**Total Cooking Time:** 1 hour, 50 Minutes

**Serving Size:** 4

**Ingredients:**

- 1 onion (chopped)
- 1 1/2 cup chickpea (dried)
- Oil
- Salt
- Pepper
- Turmeric
- Saffron threads (crumbled)
- Paprika (to taste)
- Cumin (to taste)
- Butter

**Instructions:**

1. Before you start, put the dried chickpeas in a bowl large enough to contain them and top it with water. Let to soak for at least 8 hours (preferably soak overnight). After this, remove the water and get rid of the skin.

2. Put the now skinned chickpeas in a pot. Add onion, salt, pepper, and oil. Pour 3 cups water and boil. Cover the pot and turn the heat. Then leave to simmer for 1 hour, 30 minutes, or until soft.

3. Now, transfer into a food processor and puree until thoroughly smooth. Add as much or little water as you need, depending on your texture preference.

4. Add more salt and pepper to season to your taste.

5. Garnish with paprika, cumin, with olive oil or butter.

6. Serve as soup, dip, or side dish with bread.

# Pan-Fried Scallops with Parsnip Purée & Pancetta Crumbs

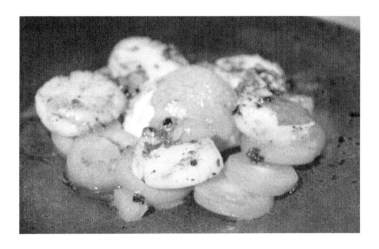

**Total Cooking Time:** 40 minutes

**Serving Size:** 4

**Ingredients:**

- 9 scallops
- 1/2 cup lemon juice
- 1 tbsp oil
- To make pancetta crumbs:
- 2 oz pancetta (cut into slices, about 5 cm)
- 1 tbsp thyme leaf (chopped)
- 2 oz fresh breadcrumb
- To make the Parsnip puree:
- 2 oz parsnip (cut)
- Butter
- 1 cup full-fat milk

**Instructions:**

**For the Pancetta crumbs:**

1. Put a big frying pan on medium heat. Put the pancetta and let it sizzle for 5 minutes, stirring occasionally. Scatter the breadcrumbs into all areas of the pan as you continue to fry and stir. When the mixture changes to brown and the crusty, transfer to a food processor. Add thyme and pulse. Transfer into an air-proof bag, especially if you are not using immediately.

**For the Parsnip puree:**

2. Put the parsnip into a pan. Add milk and bring to a boil. Bring the heat down to medium-low and leave for 15 minutes, or until the parsnips are soft. Now, pulverize in a food processor. Add butter after.

3. Grab a large frying pan, pour oil in it and heat over high heat. Season the scallops and arrange in a circle around the ends of the pan. Leave for at least 1 minute to brown them. Flip each scallop to brown the other side. After, remove the scallops and put in a plate. Now, pour the lemon juice into the pan and scrape the content at the base to make a sauce. If it is too thick, you may add water.

4. Heat the parsnip puree, and then serve into four plates. Top with the pancetta crumbs, scallops, and the juice content from the pan. Serve.

# Greek Fava Split Pea Puree

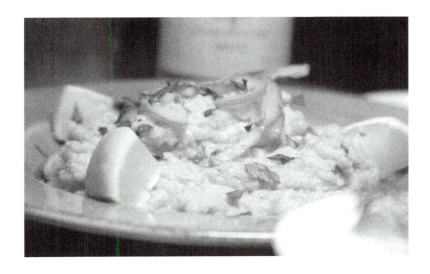

**Total Cooking Time:**

**Serving Size:**

**Ingredients:**

- 4 1/4 cup water
- 1 3/4 cups yellow split peas
- 2 tbsp olive oil
- 1 tbsp sea salt
- Additional 1/4 cup olive oil (garnish)
- 1/2 cup red onion (garnish)

**Instructions:**

1. Put the peas in a pot and add enough water to drown them. Bring to a boil and continue cooking for about 10 minutes; you should see bubbles forming. Drain and rinse the peas.

2. Get a pressure cooker and put 4 1/3 cups water and the pea. Again, bring to a boil and close. Turn the heat to low and leave to cook for 10 minutes. Fast-release pressure and open the pot.

3. In a food processor, puree the peas. Transfer back to the pot. Mix with oil and salt. Do not cover as you cook for 15 minutes over the lowest heat to transform into a thick cream. Use a wooden spoon to stir.

4. Garnish with olive oil and 1 tablespoon of diced onion. Serve.

# Smoked Aubergine Purée

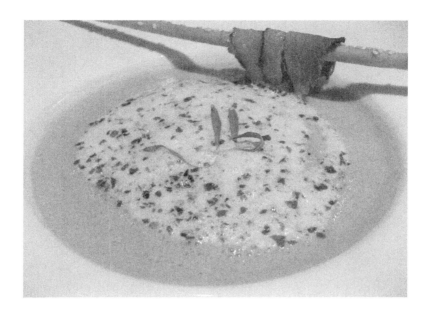

Simple description: this meal is perfect for all sorts of people. For vegetarian, it is an easy lunch, and for non-vegetarians, it goes exceptionally with grilled meat or chicken. Something for everyone, eh?

**Total Cooking Time:** 35 minutes

**Serving Size:** 4

**Ingredients:**

- 1 lemon (juiced)
- 2 aubergines
- 3 cloves garlic (crushed)
- 1 bunch dill (leaves chopped)
- 2 cup yogurt

**Instructions:**

1. Set the grill up to high heat. Cut the aubergines into half lengthways. Put on the grill for 25 minutes, or until they become tender. Ensure that you turn at intervals.

2. Afterwards, take the aubergines off the grill and leave them to cool down.

3. With a spoon, get the soft flesh out of the skin and put in a bowl. Puree the content with a fork till you get a thick mash. Pour the lemon juice and garlic and beat. Now, add the dill and yogurt.

# Creamy Corn Soup

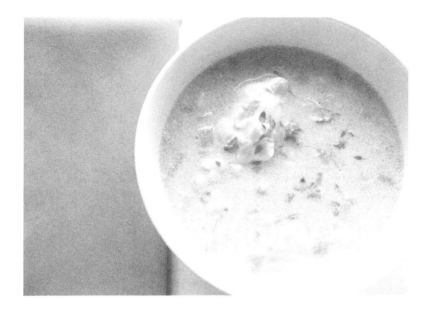

This simple cornmeal comes with loads of health benefits accompanied by a creamy taste. You prepare your ingredients in the oven before you transfer to a blender or food processor to puree.

**Total Cooking Time:** 29 minutes

**Serving Size:** 12 cups

**Ingredients:**

- 1 cup onion (diced)
- 6 cups corn kernels
- 1/2 cup celery (chopped)
- 1 ½ lbs. potatoes (diced)
- ¼ cup olive oil
- 4 cups vegetable broth
- 4 cloves garlic
- 1 tbsp maple syrup
- 1 tsp salt
- 1 tsp black pepper
- ½ cup bell pepper (diced)
- 1 tbsp fresh thyme leaves

**Instructions:**

1. First, preheat oven to 425 F. Mix the onions, corn kernels, potatoes, celery, garlic, bell pepper with the oil. Add black pepper, salt, and thyme.

2. Place the mixture on a baking sheet, preferably in an even layer. Put in the oven for 20 minutes.

3. Afterward, move the mixture to a food processor or a blender.

4. Put maple syrup and vegetable broth. Blend till you have your puree. You may have to do this in batches, depending on the capacity of your blender or food processor.

5. Serve.

6. Refrigerate leftovers and consume within 3 days.

# Strawberry Puree

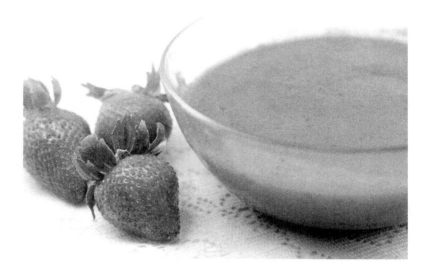

What better way is there to put your strawberries to good use than making them into a puree? This is especially useful when the strawberries are going out of season. Strawberry puree ensures that you have every bit of strawberry goodness for as long as three months if you preserve it correctly.

And by the way, does strawberry combine well with desserts? You can bet that they do!

**Total Cooking Time:** 5 minutes

**Serving Size:** 8

**Ingredients:**

- 4 cups of strawberries (hulled and halved)
- 1/4 cup sugar
- 1 tsp lemon juice

**Instructions:**

1. Pour the strawberries in a food processor or a blender. Add the lemon juice and sugar. Puree for a minute.

2. To get a smoother puree, scrape the sides of the bowl to get the content that may have been splashed. Puree for another minute or until you get a smooth mixture.

3. Pour into an air-proof container and keep in the refrigerator.

# Carrot & Star Anise Purée

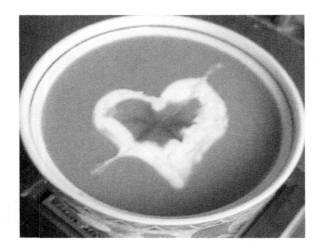

How much do you like trying out (new) things? Very much, I would like to guess. Very well then, this recipe should interest you. It will give you something new, and maybe different to add to your meal table on Christmas or any other holiday.

Personally, I think this puree is great with beef or salmon. Use moderately, though, because I have found out that the taste is quite strong. Nonetheless, this takes nothing from how much of a delight it is.

**Total Cooking Time:** 45 minutes

**Serving Size:** 8

**Ingredients:**

- 3 tbsp butter
- 2 lbs. carrots (peeled and sliced)
- 1 handful tarragon leaves
- 4 star anise
- 2 cup vegetable or chicken stock
- 1 cup double cream
- 1 lemon (juiced)

**Instructions:**

1. Put butter in a pan and melt over medium heat. Put the tarragon leaves, star anise, and carrots. Cook over low heat for 10 minutes, until the tender becomes a tad tender.

2. Add the broth and bring to a boil. Simmer for 20 minutes to cook the mixture.

3. Now, add the cream and bring to a boil again. Simmer for another minute.

4. Take the pan off the heat and remove the star anise. Pour the lemon juice and stir as you do so. Add seasoning as you like.

5. Transfer to a blender or food processor and blitz until smooth.

6. Reheat. Then serve.

# Bacon-Wrapped Scallops with Corn Puree

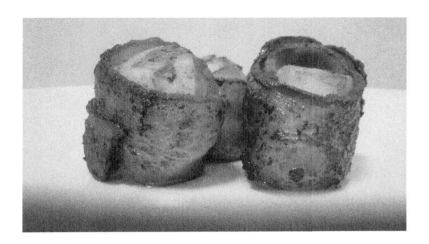

This bacon and cream meal is the perfect thing to serve to guest (of course, you can eat from it too. The best thing about is that it takes approximately 30 minutes to cook. Look at that!

**Total Cooking Time:** 30 minutes

**Serving Size:** 4

**Ingredients:**

- 1/2 lb. bacon (2 scallops take 1 slice of bacon. Cut each slice in half)
- 1 lb. scallops
- 3 cloves garlic (minced)
- 1 cup corn
- 1/2 cup cilantro fresh
- Salt
- Black Pepper
- 1 tbsp oil
- Cooking Spray

**Instructions:**

1. Preheat oven to 400 F.

2. Coat the top and bottom of the scallops with salt. Line a plate or cutting board with paper towels and put the scallop on it. Line another layer of paper towels on the scallops. Set aside.

3. Put a cast-iron pan over the stove and set heat to medium. Put the half-slices of bacon in the pan and cook. Turn as you cook until the color changes to light-brown but not long enough to turn crisp. Take off the pan and put on a plate lined with paper towels. (You may have to do this step in batches, depending on the capacity of your pan.)

4. Let the bacon cool down before touching to avoid burning your fingers. After they are cool enough, cover each scallop in 1 half-slice of bacon and lock with a toothpick.

5. Line a sheet pan with cooking oil (you can substitute with parchment paper). Put the scallops on it.

6. Put in the oven for 7-10 minutes, or until the scallops are hard and firm, and the color is white.

7. Meanwhile, proceed to make the corn puree when the scallop is cooking. Put the pan on the stove, add oil and set heat to medium.

8. Put corn and cook for some minutes. Add salt and pepper to season. Then, add garlic and cook for an extra minute. Take off the stove and leave to cool.

9. Move the mixture to a blender or food processor. Include cream. Now, Pulse until you get a rough puree. Pour the mixture back into the pan and set the heat to medium-low. Heat again.

10. Spread corn puree on each plate with a rubber spatula. Put 4-5 scallops on each plate. Garnish with fresh herbs (cilantro, basil, or parsley). Enjoy.

# Herb-Crusted Rack of Lamb with The White Bean Purée'

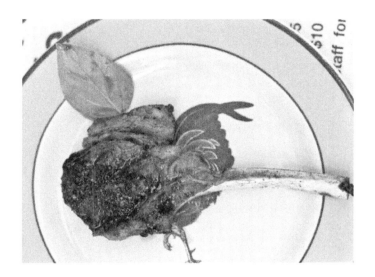

You learn to cook to have something to be proud of and exhibit at every chance you get. Now, with this lamb and bean puree recipe, you can do exactly that. It's not the easiest recipe you will find, but it's totally worth it.

**Total Cooking Time:** 50 minutes

**Serving Size:** 4

**Ingredients:**

- 2 tbsp rosemary leaves
- 2 tbsp thyme leaf
- 2 oz fresh white breadcrumb
- 2 tbsp parsley (roughly chopped)
- 2 tbsp olive oil
- 1 zest lemon
- 1 oz grated parmesan
- 1 oz Dijon mustard
- 2 x 8-bone racks of lamb( trimmed)
- 2 tbsp Dijon mustard
- 8 oz spinach leaves
- To make the bean puree:
- 1 garlic glove (chopped)
- Rosemary sprig (leaves cut/chopped)
- 6 anchovy filets
- 2 cups can butter bean (drained and rinsed)
- 1 lemon (juiced)
- 8 tbsp of extra-virgin olive oil

**Instructions:**

1. Preheat oven to 400 F.

2. Get a food processor; put the breadcrumbs, zest lemon, and Parmesan. Add 1 tbsp oil. Blitz.

3. Pour the remaining oil in a pan. Add seasoning to the lamb to your taste, then fry all sides until brown before you take off the heat. Place the rack so that the fat side is up, then coat with mustard.

4. Get the crust and the lamb and put in the oven to roast for 25 minutes or until the crust color changes to golden and the lamb is done. Put the lamb on a board to rest.

5. Meanwhile, put the beans, garlic. Anchovy fillets, rosemary, lemon juice, and seasoning and 7 tbsp olive oil into a food processor. Blitz to puree. Transfer to a pan to heat.

6. Pour the remaining oil in a new frying pan, put the spinach in it and leave to wilt. Now, back to the lamb; cut it into chop when it's rested. You have to be careful how you do this, though, to keep the crust intact.

7. Share the reheated bean puree between four plates, put some spinach on each plate, and place 3 lamb chops on each serving. You can garnish with crumbs and olive oil.

# Slow Cooker Creamy Corn Chowder

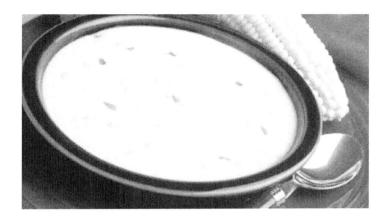

This meal is perfect for any time during the year. And it gives you a lot of room to improvise and let your creativity come to the peak. And also, you need a slow cooker to pull this off, so if you are looking to have it for dinner, you have to start in the morning. That said; this meal is sumptuous and filled with nutrients.

**Total Cooking Time:** 8 hours, 20 minutes

**Serving Size:** 6

**Ingredients:**

- 3 potatoes (chopped)
- 1 onion (chopped)
- 2 cans (about 16 oz) whole kernel corn
- 1/2 tsp kosher salt (to taste)
- 2 cups whole milk
- 1 tsp butter
- Black pepper (to taste)
- 2 cups chicken broth

**Instructions:**

1. Put the potatoes, corn, onion, chicken broth, salt, and pepper in a slow cooker and mix. Cover the mixture and cook over low heat from 7 to 9 hours.

2. Afterward, transfer to a food processor or blender. Puree to a smooth mixture.

3. Move the pureed mixture to the pot. Add milk and butter, stirring the pot as you do so.

4. Return the cover and cook over high heat for at least 30 additional minutes.

5. Serve and enjoy.

# Cauliflower Puree

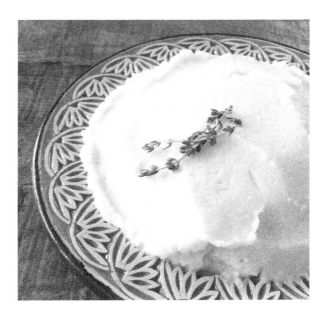

If you want something more than mashed potatoes, then cauliflower puree is for you. This may be hard to believe, but lots of people are beginning to favor cauliflower, and that means that it might just be the time for you to discover the unlimited treat it promises.

**Total Cooking Time:**

**Serving Size:**

**Ingredients:**

- 4 tbsp butter
- 1 cauliflower (cored and broken into florets)
- 1/2 tsp salt
- 1/2 cup chicken stock

**Instructions:**

1. Put the cauliflower and butter in a pot. Add the chicken stock.

2. Put over heat and bring to a boil. Remove the cover and continue to cook to over medium-high heat for 30 minutes or until most of the water is gone and the cauliflower has started to caramelize.

3. Transfer to immersion or traditional blender and puree to a smooth texture. Add salt to taste.

4. Serve.

# Pea Puree

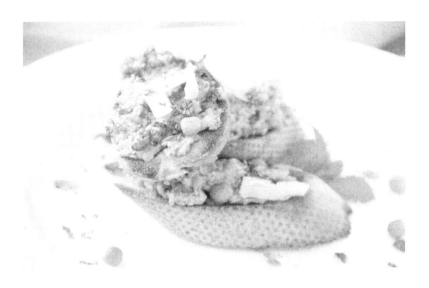

Peas give you a healthy meal option, and they can be found at any time during the year. So, why don't you try this pea puree recipe out?

**Total Cooking Time:** 20 minutes

**Serving Size:** 4

**Ingredients:**

- 1 1/2 cup frozen peas
- 1/3 cup water
- 2 tbsp unsalted butter
- 1/4 tsp salt
- 1 tsp fresh lemon juice
- 1 tbsp finely chopped onion
- 1 tbsp parsley (chopped)
- 1 tbsp tarragon
- Black pepper (ground)
- Olive oil

**Instructions:**

1. Pour water in a pot and put the peas. Cook over medium-high heat. When it softens, add salt, pepper, and butter.

2. Transfer to a food processor and puree to the desired texture. If you want it to be creamier, add a bit of olive oil.

3. Afterward, add the tarragon, parsley, onion, and fresh lemon juice.

# Potato Puree

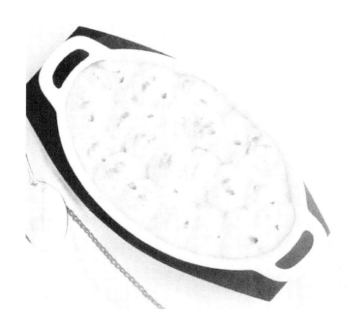

This is one simple puree recipe, featuring potatoes and some garlic for an amazing flavor for everyone to enjoy.

**Total Cooking Time:** 25 minutes

**Serving Size:** 4

**Ingredients:**

- 1 lb. potato (peeled and cut)
- 4 tbsp unsalted butter
- 2 garlic cloves
- 1/4 cup cream
- Salt
- Black Pepper

**Instructions:**

1. Pour water into a medium pot. Put the potatoes and garlic. Bring to a boil and cook over medium-high heat for 12 minutes, or until the potatoes soften.

2. Drain the water. Mash the potatoes and garlic until smooth. Add butter and continue mashing. Now, add cream and mix.

3. Season with salt and pepper to taste.

4. Serve hot and enjoy.

# Puree Meals for Babies

Here we are in the baby section. It is time to introduce your baby to solid food, isn't it? Of course, pureeing the food into smooth textures is the best way to start. The recipes in this section incorporate a blend of fruits, nuts, and vegetables. Rest assured, your baby will like them. It's going to be a perfect introduction. However, make sure that you know your family history with allergies before you use any of the ingredients.

Fair warning; you may need to keep leftovers out of grownup's reach :D.

# Spinach, Sweet Potato & Yellow Split Pea Purée

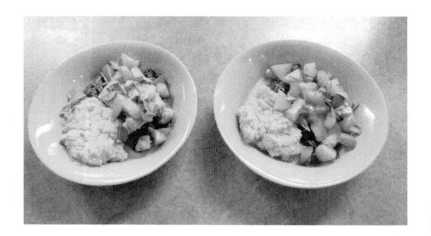

This sweet potato, split peas and spinach combination is something to serve your baby before you start them off on solids.

**Total Cooking Time:** 50 minutes

**Ingredients:**

- 2 tbsp yogurt
- 1 potato
- 5 oz yellow split peas (washed and rinsed)
- 2 oz baby leaf spinach
- Butter

**Instructions:**

1. Heat oven to 400 F. Place the potato on a baking tray and push into the oven. Roast for 45 minutes, or until tender.

2. As the potato roasts, Put a saucepan on the stove and set to medium heat. Add the butter and heat. Put the spinach, stirring the pot as you do so. Cook for 2 minutes.

3. Take the saucepan off the heat. Put the split peas and add water to sink the content.

4. Bring to a boil and cook for 10 minutes. Reduce the heat and simmer for an extra 30 minutes.

5. Take off the heat and drain. Transfer the food processor or blender. Add yogurt and spinach.

6. Go back to the potato and cut into two. Scrape out the flesh from the skin with a knife or spoon and put into the processor or blender.

7. Pulse to combine and puree the contents.

8. Serve and keep leftovers refrigerated.

# Cauliflower Cheese Purée

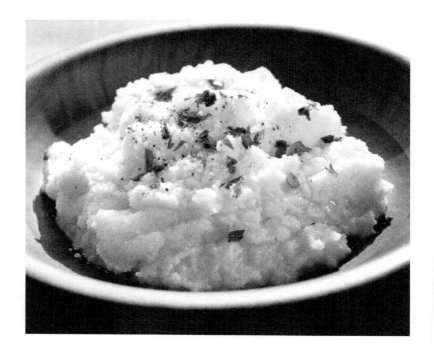

**Total Cooking Time:** 20 Minutes

**Ingredients:**

- 1/8 cup cheddar (grated)
- 1 small cauliflower (cut)
- Baby's milk

**Instructions:**

1. Put the cut cauliflower into a streamer filled with simmering water. Cook for 10 minutes, or until soft.

2. Let the cauliflower cool down, but not totally cold. When it is warm, transfer to a food processor. Add cheese and some baby milk. Blitz to get your puree.

3. Serve what you need. Keep the rest in small containers and put in the refrigerator.

# Carrot, Celeriac & Apple Purée

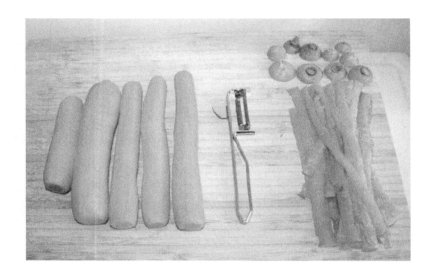

**Total Cooking Time:** 30 Minutes

**Ingredients:**

- 2 medium apples (peeled, cored, and cut)
- 3 carrots (peeled and cut)
- 5 oz celeriac (peeled and cut)
- Baby's milk

**Instructions:**

1. Place the apples, carrot, and celeriac in a steamer and put over boiling water. Let is simmer for 15 minutes.

2. Transfer to a food processor. Add milk to the mixture. Blitz to a puree.

3. Serve. Keep the leftovers refrigerated.

# Haddock, Cauliflower & Potato Purée

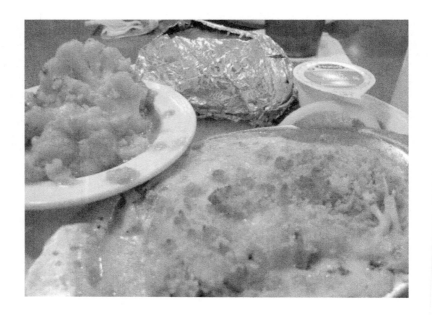

**Total Cooking Time:** 1 hour, 35 minutes

**Ingredients:**

- 5 oz haddock fillet
- 1 medium-sized potato
- 1/2 small cauliflower (cut into florets)
- Baby milk

**Instructions:**

1. Preheat oven to 400 F. Cover the potato with a foul and put on a baking tray. Place the tray in the oven and roast for 1 hour 15 minutes. Now, wrap the fillets in another foil and put on the same tray the potato is. Cook for an additional 10 minutes.

2. While it is cooking, pour water into a pan and bring to a boil. Put a steamer over it and steam the cauliflower for 8-10 minutes, or until tender.

3. When the potato is cooked, cut into half and scrape the flesh out. Turn to the fish and remove bones and skin.

4. Put the potato, cauliflower, fish, and a splash of milk into a processor. Blitz to puree.

5. Serve and refrigerate leftovers.

# Apple & Beetroot Purée

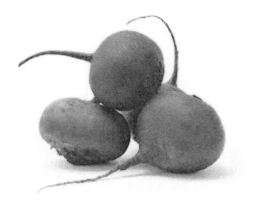

**Total Cooking Time:** 35 minutes

**Ingredients:**

- 2 apples (peeled. Cored and cut pieces)
- 1 beetroot (peeled and cut into pieces)
- Baby's milk

**Instructions:**

1. Get a steamer and put the beetroot in it. Place the steamer over boiling water and cook for 15 minutes. Now, put the apple and cool for additional 8-10 minutes, or until they are tender.

2. Transfer to the bowl of a food processor. Add the milk and blitz to puree. Get whatever content splashes to the sides of the bowl back inside while blitzing to make sure the texture of your puree is consistent.

3. Serve. Put the rest in small containers and keep refrigerated.

# Salmon, Pea & Potato Purée

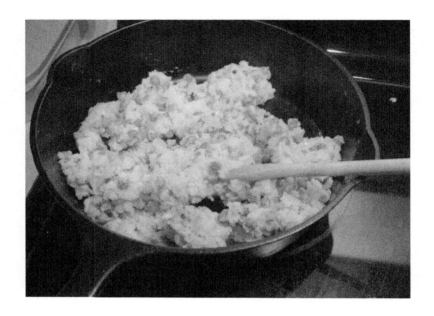

**Total Cooking Time:** 1 hour, 35 minutes

**Ingredients:**

- 1 baking potato
- 1 salmon fillet
- 2 oz peas
- Butter

**Instructions:**

1. Preheat oven to 400F.

2. Cover the potato in a foil and put on the baking tray. Put the baking tray in the oven for an hour and 15 minutes. Now, cover the fish in a foil and put on the tray too and cook for 10-15 minutes.

3. While the potato and fish are booking, pour the peas in the boiling water and leave for 3-5 minutes, or until they become soft. Drain to remove the water.

4. When the potato is ready, cut it into two halves and get the flesh out of the skin. Also, get the bones and skin out of the fish.

5. Put the potato, fish, and peas in a food processor. Add the butter (baby milk is an alternative). Blitz to puree.

6. Serve what you need. To preserve the leftovers; pour them into the small containers and then keep in the refrigerator.

# Carrot and Red Lentil Puree

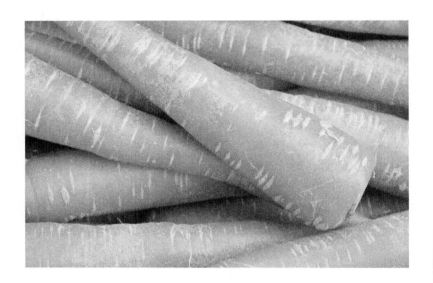

**Total Cooking Time:** 25 minutes

**Ingredients:**

- 2 oz red split lentils (rinsed)
- 4 carrots (peeled and cut)
- 2 tbsp yogurt
- 1/4 tsp ground coriander

**Instructions:**

1. Put butter in a pan and heat over medium heat. Add the coriander and leave to cook for 1 minute. Put in the lentils and carrots, stirring the mixture as you put them in.

2. Add enough water to cover the mixture and bring to a boil. Let it cook for 10 minutes before you turn the heat down. Now, simmer for 5 minutes, or until the carrots and lentils become softer.

3. Remove from the water and put in a food processor. Add yogurt and pulse until you get a smooth puree.

4. Serve and keep the leftovers frozen/refrigerated.

# Roasted Butternut Squash and Garlic Purée

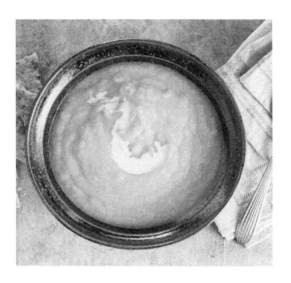

**Total Cooking Time:** 1 hour, 15 minutes

**Ingredients:**

- 1 garlic clove (with the skin)
- 1 butternut squash
- Butter or Baby milk

**Instructions:**

1. Heat oven to 400 F. Put the butternut on a baking sheet and wrap with a foil. Put in the oven and roast for 45 minutes. Put the garlic beside the butternut and roast for an additional 15 minutes.

2. Leave the butternut and garlic to cool before you handle. Get the flesh out of the butternut squash and get rid of the seeds and skin. Get the garlic out of the skin too.

3. Transfer the butternut and garlic to a food processor and pulse to a puree. If the puree is too thick, add butter or baby milk to loosen.

# Banana and Avocado Puree

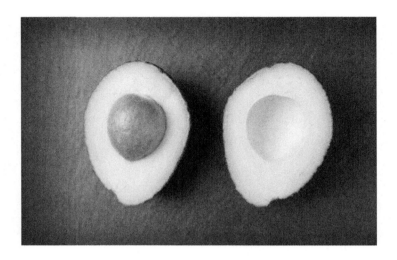

**Total Cooking Time:** 5 minutes

**Ingredients:**

- 1/2 small ripe banana
- 1/2 small ripe avocado
- 1 tbsp yogurt

**Instructions:**

1. Cut the avocado into two halves, take off the stone and get the flesh out the center; put in a bowl.

2. Put the banana in the bowl too. With a spoon, mash the content to a puree.

3. Add the yogurt and stir consistently.

4. Serve.

# Spiced Pear Purée

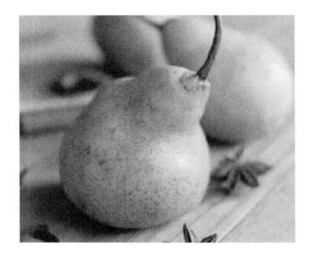

**Total Cooking Time:** 10 minutes

**Ingredients:**

- 2 pears (peeled, cored and cut)
- A pinch of cinnamon
- Baby's milk

**Instructions:**

1. Get a steamer and put the pear in it. Place the steamer over simmering water. Cook for 8 minutes, or until soft.

2. Put in a food processor. Add a pinch of cinnamon. Blitz to a puree. While you are it, add some baby milk to ensure a smooth texture.

3. Serve what you need and keep the leftover in small containers and keep them refrigerated.

# Rice Puree and Spiced Carrot

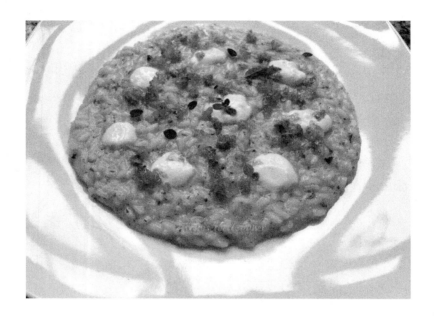

**Total Cooking Time:** 50 minutes

**Ingredients:**

- 2 carrot (chopped)
- 1 1/2 cups water
- 1/4 tsp cumin
- 1/2 tsp dried parsley
- 1/2 cup of short-grain brown rice

**Instructions:**

1. Pour water and rice into a pot. Put on the stove and bring to a boil.

2. Turn the heat to low. Then cover the pot and leave to simmer for about 30 minutes.

3. Put the carrots into the pot and let it cook for an extra 15 minutes. Ensure that you still have some water left in the pot, to ensure you have a smooth puree.

4. Move the content to a food processor. Add cumin and parsley. Puree. Add water if it is too thick.

5. Serve.

# Mango Blueberry Puree with A Splash Of Milk

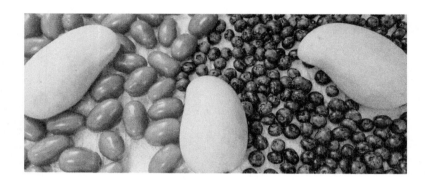

**Total Cooking Time:** 1 minute

**Ingredients:**

- 1 Banana
- 1/2 mango (peeled and diced)
- 1/2 cup baby milk
- 1/2 cup blueberries

**Instructions:**

1. Put banana, mango, and blueberries in a food processor. Add milk. Puree until smooth.

2. Serve.

# Banana Puree & Roast Pear

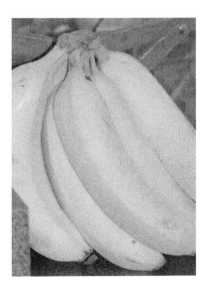

**Total Cooking Time:** 30 minutes

**Ingredients:**

- 2 pears (peeled and cut)
- 2 Bananas (peeled and cut)

**Instructions:**

1. First, heat oven to 400 F.

2. Put the cut bananas and eats on a baking sheet or parchment paper. Roast in the oven for 23-25 minutes.

3. Transfer to a food processor or blender and puree until smooth.

4. Pour into a bowl to cool down

5. Serve.

# Apple Walnut Puree

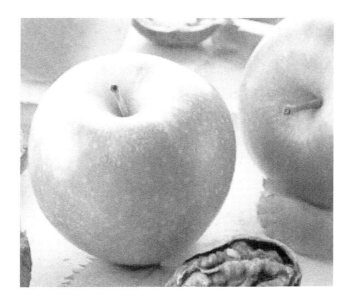

**Total Cooking Time:** 12 minutes

**Ingredients:**

- 1/4 cup walnuts (remove the shells and cut into halves)
- 2 apples (peeled and cored)
- 1/8 tsp cinnamon

**Instructions:**

1. Put walnuts and apples in a steamer and place on boiling water.

2. Cook for 10 minutes to soften the apples; pierce with a fork to make sure of this.

3. Transfer the apple and walnut to a food processor. Take 3 tablespoons of water from the pot and add to the food processor. Also, add the cinnamon.

4. Puree until smooth.

5. Pour into a bowl to cool. Then serve.

# Banana and Strawberry Puree

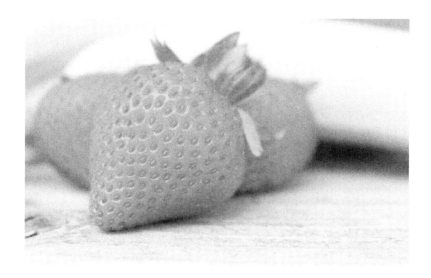

**Total Cooking Time:** 5 minutes

**Ingredients:**

- 1 medium banana (peeled and cut)
- 3 strawberries (washed and leaves removed)
- Baby's milk

**Instructions:**

1. Put the banana pieces and strawberries in a food processor or blender.

2. Puree until smooth. As you puree, add baby's milk to ensure uniform consistency.

3. Serve and refrigerate leftovers.

# Conclusion

Well, well, well, here we are, at the end of this book. I wish there was more, but there isn't. Thank you for coming on this journey with me; I'm sure you have learned a lot. I mean, I would certainly hope so.

This book is yours, so free feel to consult at any time. I hope you get the best out of this book and enjoy every step as much as I enjoyed writing it.

Cheers!

# About the Author

Molly Mills always knew she wanted to feed people delicious food for a living. Being the oldest child with three younger brothers, Molly learned to prepare meals at an early age to help out her busy parents. She just seemed to know what spice went with which meat and how to make sauces that would dress up the blandest of pastas. Her creativity in the kitchen was a blessing to a family where money was tight and making new meals every day was a challenge.

Molly was also a gifted athlete as well as chef and secured a Lacrosse scholarship to Syracuse University. This was a blessing to her family as she was the first to go to college and at little cost to her parents. She took full advantage of her college education and earned a business degree. When she graduated, she joined her culinary skills and business acumen into a successful catering business. She wrote her first e-book after a customer asked if she could pay for several of her recipes. This sparked the entrepreneurial spirit in Mills and she thought if one person wanted them, then why not share the recipes with the world!

Molly lives near her family's home with her husband and three children and still cooks for her family every chance she gets. She plays Lacrosse with a local team made up of her old teammates from college and there are always some tasty nibbles on the ready after each game.

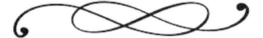

# Don't Miss Out!

Scan the QR-Code below and you can sign up to receive emails whenever Molly Mills publishes a new book. There's no charge and no obligation.

Printed in Great Britain
by Amazon

80934419R00048